EYE CARE
Naturally

A Guide to Prevention and Natural Treatment
of Common Eye Conditions.

2nd Edition

March, 2004

By
E. Michael Geiger, O.D.

Eye Care *Naturally*

E. Michael Geiger, O.D.

Cover design by Dianne Cooper Bridges

ISBN 1-884820-72-7
Library of Congress Catalog Card Number 2002116691
1. Eye 2. Health 3. Medicine 4. Natural Health 5.Optometry

Printed in USA

Safe Goods Publishing
561 Shunpike Rd.
Sheffield, MA 01257
413-229-7935

FOREWORD

This book provides the reader with an understanding of some common eye afflictions that affect, or will affect, most of us including our relatives and friends. Conditions covered include cataracts, glaucoma, macular degeneration, retinitis pigmentosa, diabetic retinopathy, styes, dry eye, red eye and computer eyestrain. This book is not intended to be technical in nature, but rather is written in larger, easy-to-read type as an easy-to-understand concise guide that can give you alternatives to surgery or drug treatment. Information is presented to dispel misinformation about eye conditions. For example: cataracts are not a "skin growing over the eye" as many believe; glaucoma is not glucoma, as often mispronounced. If you desire more technical information, please research more detailed information at your local library or on the Internet.

Eye Care Naturally provides the reader with suggestions on how he or she may be able to avoid some specific eye afflictions, postponing their occurrence, or treating them in a nonmedical fashion. Many physicians tell their patients that, "there is nothing that can be done for your condition." They continue to advise that the only course of action is to wait for the eventual surgery or even blindness. They are advised to return for an eye checkup in three months, or six months, so the doctor can determine how much vision has been lost. In the opinion of the author, this is nonsense! Wait and do nothing except worry about the inevitable?

The author's words give hope and an alternative plan of action to avoid or at least delay "the inevitable." The author is not suggesting that the reader use this information to replace medical treatment where such treatment exists, but rather to utilize this information as an adjunct to supplement medical care. The author repeatedly cautions the reader to check with his or her physician, prior to following any of the recommendations cited. Discuss your concerns with your eye physician and share our techniques with them.

Many people who buy this book will do so because they want to avoid or treat a specific concern. Although each is covered in a separate chapter, the author advises that you read *Eye Care Naturally* in its entirety. He stresses that useful information in every chapter may apply to conditions cited in other chapters.

The author, Dr. E. Michael Geiger, has been a practicing optometrist for over forty years. He has written many optometric articles and booklets for publication. He is a past president of the Queens County Optometric Society. Dr. Geiger became interested in nutrition and how proper diet affects not only the body as a whole but specifically the eyes. Dr. Geiger has studied and researched vast information on nutrition and the role it plays in vision. He has discussed this subject with nutritionists, and with optometrists who incorporate nutrition into their practices.

Dr. Geiger has extensively surveyed numerous nutritional supplement companies that make claims about their products and eye care. Some supplements he favors above similar ones on the market. If you would like further information on these products you can contact Dr. Geiger directly.

-Dr. Joseph Y. Bistricer

Contact information:
E. Michael Geiger, O.D.
E-mail: pure4us@aol.com

TABLE OF CONTENTS

Chapter 1

CATARACTS

Cataracts are the most common condition affecting our eyes as we age. They are the leading cause of blindness in the world. Popular opinion holds the myth that cataracts will affect all of us if we live long enough, much like graying hair. Some of us develop cataracts at a relatively early age, yet there are people in their nineties that have no sign of cataracts at all. Statistics show that most of us will develop age-related cataracts in our sixties and seventies. I believe that we do not have to become part of the statistics and develop cataracts, as I will outline in this chapter.

There are many different types and causes of cataracts that can occur at any age, but we will focus on those cataracts that form gradually as a by-product of the aging process. These are termed senile cataracts and normally affect two out of three people over the age of seventy.

WHAT ARE CATARACTS?

Inside the eye there is a structure called the crystalline lens. It is clear—like a clear marble—and changes shape to focus the light entering the eye onto the back of the eye (the retina). This is how our eyes change focus from far to near and let's us still see clearly. The most commonly accepted theory is that as we age, the crystalline lens loses its flexibility. That is why we need reading glasses or bifocals to read with, generally when we get into our forties. Our ability to focus at near print and objects decreases. In addition to losing its flexibility, the crystalline lens starts to lose its clarity. Just as the white of an egg goes from clear to white as we heat the egg, so does the lens within our eye go from clear to white. That is a cataract.

When the white of the lens is too dense for light to pass through it, and we cannot see clearly, the lens can be removed from our eye surgically and a new clear plastic lens can be inserted in its place. This is referred to as cataract surgery, and the new lens is known as an implant or an IOL. Some eyes are not suitable for an IOL. The alternative is to wear cataract eyeglasses or contact lenses.

Cataracts are believed to be caused by a life-time of exposure to the ultraviolet rays of the sun. The UV rays actually can cause a "slow boil" of the lens. It may also be caused by poor nutrition, or by an accumulation of sugars in the lens found in people who have diabetes. In addition to these causes cataracts could occur from protein changes in the lens due to oxidation. Oxidation is what causes iron to rust and cut apples to turn brown. Heavy smokers and people who live in sunny climates seem to be more prone to developing cataracts at an earlier age than nonsmokers and people who live in areas where there is not as much sunlight.

When your eye doctor tells you that you are developing cataracts, it does not mean that you are going to require surgery any time soon. It means that you should be aware of the reasons that things may not appear as clear or as bright to you as they once did. You may need extra light when reading or experience excessive glare from sunlight or on-coming headlights. You require surgery when your eyesight interferes with your normal way of life.

However, be aware that cataracts usually do not develop at the same rate in each eye, so you should have an annual eye exam to determine when the eye with the more advanced cataract requires surgery. Your overall health plays a role in this de-termination also, so it is wise to follow the advice of your doctor, and also to get a second opinion prior to surgery.

HOW CAN YOU PREVENT CATARACTS?

There are several things that you can do to help prevent the early formation of cataracts. The simplest is to keep the sun out of your eyes. Wear a hat with a brim to shade your eyes or sunglasses that block *all* of the UV rays. These are available at any optical shop. If you buy sunglasses from a non-optical shop, like a department store or a drug store, you may not get sunglasses that block all of the harmful UV rays. UV rays can penetrate clouds, so it is a good idea to wear UV blocking lenses whenever you are outdoors in daylight. UV block can be applied professionally to clear prescription eyeglasses, and is a very good investment to help retard cataract formation.

You can also help prevent the early formation of cataracts with proper nutrition by eating the right foods. Foods that support eye health (and your general health also) include:

- all kinds of green vegetables, garlic, carrots, onions, corn, and yams.
- citrus fruit, cantaloupe, and apples.
- sea vegetables, seeds, almonds, and whole grains, which are valuable for their content of Vitamin E and other antioxidants.

Antioxidants are extremely important in assisting the body in preventing the formation of cataracts.[1] The crystalline lens in the eye is composed primarily of proteins. These proteins are called crystallins and are what gives the lens its transparency. When these crystallins are damaged, for example by exposure to ultra-violet rays, free radicals form, which cause the crystallins to clump together. This is what is thought to cause the lens to lose its transparency—forming a cataract. Another source of free radicals is the polluted air that we breathe and our every day personal care and toiletry products that we use.

Research indicates that antioxidants attack these free radicals, therefore, it is important to have antioxidants included in our diet. Taking just one

---

[1] *AREDS* sponsored by the NEI. "The Effect of Antioxidant Vitamins and Zinc on Age-Related Macular Degeneration and Cataract." Oct. 2001

type of antioxidant (such as vitamin C or E) is not enough because there are hundreds of different types of free radicals. A variety of foods containing many different antioxidants must be eaten to counter the many different free radicals.

Foods to avoid are foods that generate free radicals such as fried, charcoal barbecued, and smoked foods. Never eat rancid oils or foods containing hydrogenated or partially hydrogenated oils (commonly found in margarine and butter substitutes). Eat butter. Never eat swordfish, which is high in mercury content. Mercury has been linked to a particular type of cataract in addition to doing other harm to your body.

Most of us are in a hurry when it comes to food and we find it difficult to eat properly. Prepared foods commonly include ingredients that may not be good for us, and lack many beneficial nutrients. The preparation of food should also be considered. What oils are being used? How is it cooked? Is it overcooked? (Beneficial enzymes necessary for digestion can be destroyed by the cooking process, therefore, proper nutrient absorption may be compromised.)

Read labels and ask questions. Has the food been exposed to free-radical generating chemicals and pesticides? What chemicals are in the feed of the beef or chicken that you eat, and which drugs have the animals been injected with? Free-range, drug-free meat or fowl and organically grown fruits and vegetables may be a better choice. The ability to eat properly is not an easy task nowadays. It can be done, but it does require effort.

SUPPLEMENTS

Today we are fortunate to have available to us supplements that replace the nutrients deficient in our food.

Number one in importance in my estimation is a well-rounded multi-vitamin and mineral supplement. Pay particular attention to the mineral content because you obtain very little from food. Since most bottled or city water has the minerals removed through the purification process, adding a vitamin/mineral supplement to your dietary regime is essential. You will want to purchase a preparation containing multiple essential vitamins, essential and trace minerals, amino acid chelates, and enzymes, all of which support proper nutritional needs. My favorite also contains important antioxidants. Also important is a multi-vitamin/mineral supplement for people fifty and older. It is formulated for aging systems which have different requirements. Most manufacturers just list their ingredients, but neglect to describe their potential for absorption by the cells of the body. I have investigated this from various manufacturers and have my favorites. So should you.

In my opinion a supplement that contains ingredients specifically to support vision and ocular health should be part of your daily regimen. Many are available, but make sure that the one you use contains, at least, these ingredients: lutein, bilberry, eyebright, quercetin, selenium, zinc, Vitamins C and E and beta carotene.

The antioxidants are important to neutralize free radicals and help prevent cataract formation, or slow down its development. I advise selecting a very broad-spectrum army of super antioxidants that has the ability to change and combat a variety of free radicals. Also, there are now powerful new detoxification products that can assist the body in getting rid of toxins that we take in through the foods that we eat and the environment that we live in.

Several studies of people with cataracts have been performed, notably one at the University of Western Ontario[2] and one in Finland.[3] These studies found that people who did not include antioxidant supplements in their diets had a much higher incidence of developing cataracts than those who did include antioxidants in their diet. A broad-spectrum antioxidant formulated specifically for eyes is your best bet for neutralizing the greatest number of free radicals that cause cataract formation.

I recommend taking garlic tablets to aid in blood circulation. Co-enzyme Q10 is the last supplement that might retard cataract formation or slow down its progression. Q10 is especially

[2] Robertson J., Donner A., Trevithick J., "A Possible Role for Vitamins C and E in Cataract Prevention," *Amer J of Clinical Nutr,* Vol 53 (Suppl), pp. 346S-51S, 1991.
[3] Rouhiainen R., Rouhiainen H., Salonen J., "Association Between Low Plasma Vitamin C Concentration and Progression of Early Cortical Lens Opacities." *Amer J of Epidem.* Vol. 144, pp. 496-500, 1996.

beneficial when combined with Vitamin E, which work as energy converters for enzyme depleted systems, nourish the heart muscle, assist with circulation and provide the body with more energy.

To summarize cataract prevention, wear proper ultra-violet protection for your eyes, eat the proper foods, avoid the foods that can harm you, and take your supplements. By following this simple regimen, you are likely to help delay cataract formation, and you are likely to help slow down or halt its progression if you already have cataracts. In some cases, the cataract that has formed may reverse and eyesight in that eye may improve.

Always consult with a physician knowledgeable in nutrition before radically changing your diet and before taking any new supplements. You could possibly have a condition that would be aggravated by these recommendations or be contraindicated when used in conjunction with specific medications. Be consumer savvy when purchasing supplements. Many brands marketed may not contain the exact ingredients as listed on the bottle. If you want to be sure that you are getting what you are paying for, contact the manufacturer and ask questions. Your eye care professional may be well educated in nutritional protocols too, so ask him or her for a preferred list of my recommended products many of which are not sold in stores.

Chapter 2
Glaucoma

The leading cause of blindness in the United States today is glaucoma. There are several types of glaucoma, but they fall into two main categories: chronic open angle glaucoma and acute closed angle glaucoma. By far, the more common of the two is chronic open angle glaucoma. This form of glaucoma has no symptoms at the early stages, and so goes undetected in many cases until it is too late to prevent the ultimate blindness that follows. It generally is caused by a gradual increase in the fluid pressure within the eye. This increased pressure gradually destroys the cells of the optic nerve and retina leading to blindness.

What causes this gradual increase in the pressure within the eye is still unknown. The first retinal cells to deteriorate are not at the extreme periphery of the retina, nor are they in the very center, so central vision remains sharp, and peripheral vision remains normal. This in-between "doughnut" area gradually expands, and the last to be affected is the central vision. That is why glaucoma is asymptomatic until it is too late. The nerve cells that were destroyed cannot be brought back to life again.

Another form of chronic open angle glaucoma is where the eye pressure remains low or normal, and yet the optic nerve cells and the retinal cells start to deteriorate in the same manner as described above. This is more difficult to detect and requires special testing.

Glaucoma can develop at any age, but chronic open angle glaucoma is more likely to occur after the age of forty, and most likely to occur after the age of sixty. Glaucoma is more prevalent among people who have a family history of the disease, and among African-Americans. Your best defense against the ravages of this condition is to have an annual eye exam with a pressure test for glaucoma. This is how most of these cases are detected and if caught at an early stage, the eye pressure can usually be regulated through the use of special eye drops without any loss of vision. In some cases, more drastic methods are necessary to control the eye pressure. A visual fields test should also be performed for anyone that is in the high-risk category for glaucoma, or anyone who has the disease.

Acute closed angle glaucoma occurs very suddenly with intense pain in the eyes, and must immediately be treated with surgery. This type of glaucoma is caused by a blockage in the drainage mechanism within the eye, so the fluid that is produced cannot drain out. This causes the pressure within the eye to soar, producing extreme pain.

Treating glaucoma naturally *in addition to* the medical treatment that we are receiving, slowing down its progression, and preventive measures for those of us who are predisposed to it are all the same. We can use the same techniques as outlined in the previous chapter: proper nutrition through a healthy diet and supplementation.

GOOD NUTRITION

A balanced diet with plenty of fresh fruits and vegetables, and cold-water fish every other day, can play a large role in maintaining your general health as well as your eye health. I recommend the following protocol:

- Low-fat protein foods such as turkey, chicken, eggs, and some soy products.
- Tofu or tempe are wonderful meat substitutes.
- Whole grains (avoid most breads, rolls, cakes, and pastas on the market). Avoid white rice.
- Organic products and free-range meat and poultry from the health food store. *Note:* Many health food products are also available in your local supermarket as they are becoming more aware of the demand for organic fruits and vegetables, whole grain products, and hormone and pesticide-free chickens and turkeys.
- Almonds, sunflower seeds, cantaloupe, spinach once a week, garlic, onions, and carrots.
- Olive oil or Canola oil for cooking.

What to avoid? Caffeine. Caffeine has been found to increase eye pressure. Caffeine is found in coffee, tea, and cola drinks. Switch to a coffee substitute, herbal tea, or any noncola drink. Decaffeinated coffee is not a viable option because the decaffeinating process might cause other health issues to develop. Purified water is the best drink of all, and plenty of it should be consumed every day. However, people with glaucoma should not drink more than four to six ounces of water at a time, as too much water at one time may increase eye pressure. Rather, they should consume smaller amounts of water frequently throughout the day.

SUPPLEMENTS

- As previously mentioned in the chapter on cataracts, a good vitamin-mineral supplement is essential, not only for your eye health, but for your general well-being. My favorite has the best combination of vitamins and minerals in the form that provides maximum absorbability.
- As mentioned in the previous chapter, a supplement specific, for eyes should contain at least lutein, bilberry, eyebright, zinc, selenium, quercetin, Vitamins C and E and beta carotene.
- Good eye health can also be supported by taking an enteric coated Omega-3 fish oil capsule containing some Vitamin E. This is beneficial especially if you are not a fish eater. People who are allergic to fish, can obtain their Omega-3s from flax seed (as an oil capsule or fresh ground seed form).
- Another one from my list of essential supplements is garlic, which comes with a long list of health benefits. I recommend one whole clove a day, or an enteric-coated fresh garlic tablet that dissolves in the intestines thereby avoiding "garlic breath."

- I also recommend Ginkgo Biloba since recent studies have indicated its benefit for people with glaucoma.[4] Ginkgo, along with other supplements mentioned in this section, are recommended specifically for people with glaucoma or for people who have borderline glaucoma, or for people who are at risk for glaucoma.

Again, check with your physician before taking any nutritional supplements or changing your eating habits if you have a medical condition, are pregnant, or are taking any medication.

---

[4] Ritch R., *Med Hypotheses*, 54 (2), pp 221-35, Feb 2000; Chung H.S., et al. *J Ocular Pharmacol Ther*, 15 (3), pp 233-40, Jun 1999.

Chapter 3
Macular Degeneration

A recent study of more than 14,000 adults revealed that fewer than 1 percent under the age of 64 had AMD, but raises to 13 percent over the age of 85.[5] There are other studies that indicate an even higher percentage. Age-related macular degeneration (AMD) is the leading cause of blindness in people over the age of eighty. Not total blindness, as with glaucoma, but a loss of central vision. Peripheral vision remains intact, but those who suffer from macular degeneration cannot read, watch television, recognize people, and cannot see anything directly in front of them. People with light colored eyes may be more at risk.

The macula is the central area of the retina that is responsible for the sharpest direct vision, and for color vision. AMD can develop in people as young as fifty. There are two types of AMD. One is the "dry" type that can take years to develop. The other is the "wet" type that generally requires immediate medical intervention. The cause of macular degeneration is not known, but it is believed that there is insufficient disposal of the digested macula wastes into the bloodstream, which causes them to build up in the macular area and block the light-receiving cells. There is also a

---

[5] Ophthalmology 108: 697-704, 2001.

thinning of the pigment cells in this area. Macular degeneration has no known medical cure.

There are many doctors who say that the use of herbal supplements, vitamins, and minerals might prevent macular degeneration from occurring and may slow down its progression in people who already have the condition. Since there is no known medical cure, what does one have to lose by taking these supplements? It's a viable option.

Begin by taking to your doctor, a list of the supplements and foods that you intend to use selected from information in this book. If your doctor tells you that supplements are just a lot of hogwash, then he or she is not up to date with current literature, and I would suggest that you consult with another doctor who is informed along these lines. You must be careful about any supplement program you begin on your own. Some selections may not be good for your overall health, or can interfere with a medication that you are taking, or aggravate another medical condition.

FOOD AND SUPPLEMENTS

- Vitamin C can help prevent blood vessels in the retina from breaking, and can help prevent the growth of new blood vessels in the macula, which can interfere with vision. Foods rich in vitamin C are citrus fruits (oranges, lemons, and grapefruit), tomatoes, apricots, berries, grapes, and cherries.

- Vitamins A and D, found in cold-water fish. These include salmon, sardines, cod, and trout.
- Omega-3 fatty acids. These help prevent blood vessel clotting, a major contributing factor to macular degeneration. Found in cold-water fish, it is beneficial to include them in your diet at least every other day. Again, never eat swordfish, which is high in mercury content. Mercury can be very harmful to your eyes.
- Garlic helps prevent your blood from clotting within your vascular system. It also helps raise your HDL (good) cholesterol and lower your LDL (bad) cholesterol. Garlic can help your eyes and your body in other ways too, such as aiding in blood circulation. One clove a day should be eaten, or else an equivalent in tablet form should be taken. The form of the garlic tablet is important too, so you should check with your supplier to be assured that it is derived from fresh garlic, which is best, and that it is enteric-coated so that it avoids "garlic breath."
- Other healthful nutrients good for your eyes include fresh, dark, leafy greens, such as kale, collard greens, spinach once a week, Swiss chard, watercress, and parsley. Always buy organic whenever you can to avoid the harmful free-radical forming chemicals that are sprayed on produce and used as fertilizer in the soil that they grow in.
- Red wine: The Journal of the American Geriatric Society reported a correlation between the con-

sumption of red wine (one glass daily) and the retarded onset of age-related macular degeneration (AMD.)[6]

- The vitamin and mineral tablets or caplets that includes trace minerals I have previously mentioned is necessary for your eye and general health. The vitamin/mineral supplement should also contain enzymes as an ingredient that is essential for maximum absorption.

- A supplement specifically for eye health containing 6 to 15 mg. of lutein and zinc is essential for preventing macular degeneration. 20-40 mg. of lutein depending upon the stage of AMD is required to slow down the progression of AMD, and in some cases improves eyesight. Lutein increases macular pigment levels that protect against AMD.

- Glutathione is a universal antioxidant in the retina that may be helpful in maintaining retinal function. The liver produces a large pool of glutathione to flood diseased tissues with this antioxidant and studies have shown that it plays an important role in AMD.[7] Since older adults exhibit lower levels of glutathione it would be prudent to supplement your diet with MSM, the only form of sulfur that your body can utilize to produce glutathione.

- Genistein, a compound of soy, may be beneficial. The most visually debilitating form of AMD occurs when abnormal new blood vessels

---

[6] Jrnl of the Amer Geriatric Soc., Vol 46, pp 1-7, 1998.
[7] *Investigative Ophthalmology*, ARVO Abstracts 435, B346, 1997.

encroach on the macula and destroy it—the "wet" form of AMD. Genistein reportedly inhibits the formation of these undesirable blood vessels.[8]

- A good calcium supplement is also recommended as being essential for strong bones and as an aid in the prevention and treatment of osteoporosis. The calcium supplement should be chelated and include magnesium and Vitamin D to be properly absorbed and utilized by the body.

To support eye health, exercise (even just a twenty minute walk a day), is not only good for your heart, but by increasing your blood flow, it transports needed oxygen to your eyes and increases the removal of cellular waste, which is a critical factor in AMD. Always wear good UV-absorbing sunglasses when outdoors in daylight. Brown-tinted lenses are recommended, since they best absorb the blue rays of the spectrum, which are the most harmful to eyes with macular degeneration. Again, I advise you to check with your physician before taking any foods or supplements recommended here. They may interfere with medication that you are taking or might not be recommended for a particular condition that you have.

---

[8] *Current Eye Research* 20: pp. 215-24, 2000.

Chapter 4
Retinitis Pigmentosa

Retinitis Pigmentosa, also known as RP, is a relatively rare eye disease. About half of those afflicted with it have a family history of the disease. It manifests itself in young adults by decreasing their peripheral vision. RP progresses slowly and can eventually lead to total blindness.

What occurs is that the pigment cells of the retina, as they grow older, tend to clump together on the retina blocking light from reaching the new pigment cells that have reached maturity underneath them. In a healthy eye, the old pigment cells, as with all old cells in the body (except in the eye's crystalline lens), are transported away by the bloodstream and replaced by new cells. In RP, these old pigment cells are not carried away, but build up and clump together. There is no known medical cure for this disease.

WHAT CAN WE DO?

I am not going to suggest a cure for retinitis pigmentosa, nor am I going to suggest how to remove the clumps of pigment. I am going to describe what you can do that may slow down the progression of the disease, and how you might possibly prevent it from occurring.

Healthy bodies and eyes depend very heavily on the oxidation of its cells; that is, on the red blood cells delivering oxygen to the cells of the body and the eye. The red blood corpuscles transport oxygen to the cells, and then the cells have to have the ability to absorb the oxygen and to utilize it to stay healthy, active, and useful. One of the main ingredients of every cell in the body is glutathione, which is necessary for this oxidation process to occur. Since the body requires sulfur to manufacture glutathione, we can take supplements or eat foods that will aid the body in the production of glutathione. Many experts agree that eating properly and taking the right supplements can slow down the progression of RP and decrease your chances of it developing, especially with a family history of RP. Not only will these suggestions help your eyes, but they will aid in your overall health too.

WHAT TO EAT AND DRINK

- Eat foods rich in lutein and beta carotene, which are found in fresh vegetables.
- Try to vary your vegetables. Select different colors and different textures to derive a variety of different nutrients. I always recommend organic produce to avoid the harmful chemicals and sprays used on non-organic foods.
- Eat cold-water fish every other day. The varieties include salmon, sardines, trout, and codfish, rich

in Omega-3 and Omega-6 fatty acids (for your "good" cholesterol.)

- Cook with olive oil and use extra virgin olive oil or fresh flax seed oil on your salads and whole grain pasta. Canola oil and peanut oil are acceptable for cooking also. Avoid unsaturated and hydrogenated oils, such as found in margarine.
- Avoid refined sugar and products that contain it as well as all artificial sweeteners, such as aspartame.
- Avoid MSG (monosodium glutamate).
- Restrict your intake of refined carbohydrates.
- Eat whole grains only. Your health food store carries a large variety of whole grains. It is good to familiarize yourself with them. Avoid processed grains and processed foods in general.
- Limit your consumption of alcohol to one drink a day at most.
- Stop smoking and avoid being near people who are smoking.
- Always wear good sunglasses with UV block when outdoors during daylight. Remember, UV rays penetrate clouds.

SUPPLEMENTS

- MSM: the most important supplement to take for people with RP and for people who fear RP. MSM is the only form of sulfur that your body can utilize to produce glutathione. It does not affect people who are allergic to sulfur and is as harmless as water. MSM is found in every cell in your body. It originates in the ocean and evaporates with water to form clouds. Rain from the clouds carries the MSM to plants that readily absorb it through their root system. It is very volatile and evaporates with water very quickly, which is why it is only present in fresh, raw or lightly cooked vegetables. It is very difficult to assess just how fresh the produce that we eat is, and whether or not the absorption of MSM by the plant's root system has been interfered with by some chemical spray or fertilizer. Therefore, to be safe, I recommend taking MSM as a supplement before each meal.

- Of course a good multi-vitamin mineral supplement is essential, such as I recommended previously. For people fifty and older, I recommend a special blend designed for their age group which has different requirements than for younger people.

- Lutein, bilberry, zinc, selenium, and beta carotene combined in a supplement specific for the eyes.

- Co-enzyme Q10 is a vascular nutrient and energy converter. The best possible blood circulation with oxygen rich blood is essential to eye health and your strongest ally in slowing the progression of RP.

- Omega-3 capsules supply you with the much-needed Omega-3 found in fish oils. An alternative to fish oil is flax seed oil in capsule form, ground seed, or a liquid oil that can be found in the refrigerator of your health food store. Make sure oils are not rancid or they will do you more harm than good. Some Vitamin E in the fish oil capsule prevents rancidity.

- Capsicum fruit, otherwise known as Cayenne pepper, available in your health food store, helps to promote better circulation and oxygen absorption. It is a good RP supplement.
- Lastly I recommend a good multi-antioxidant formulated specifically for eyes. There is none that I know of that is as advanced and as progressive as the one that I have found and recommend. It contains a huge variety of antioxidants that work in tandem with each other in order to help eliminate free radicals, which can be so destructive to your eyes and general health.

Of course, as I have repeatedly advised, it is highly recommended that you consult with your physician before taking any of the foods or supplements outlined in this book. As for my specific recommendations, ask your eye doctor about them and where you might obtain them.

Chapter 5
Diabetic Retinopathy

Before addressing diabetic retinopathy, a short description of diabetes itself is necessary. There are two types of diabetes. Type 1, or insulin dependent diabetes can affect you at any age. Type 2 occurs in adults primarily, but is occurring more frequently nowadays in youngsters. It is generally controlled with oral medication, exercise, or diet. Both types of diabetes require careful attention to diet. Both types can affect the eyes causing cataracts, macular edema, and/or diabetic retinopathy. In this chapter we shall concern ourselves with diabetic retinopathy.

This condition can occur in someone who has either type of diabetes for at least five years. Five years from inception may occur a lot sooner than five years from diagnosis, so any diabetic should be wary of diabetic eye changes.

One of the earliest changes that occur in diabetics is a significant change in the refractive power of the eyes. That means a sudden change in eyesight requiring a large change in eyeglass prescription. Another symptom is sudden diplopia, or seeing double. Either of these symptoms requires a blood glucose determination. When the blood glucose level is much higher than normal due to the body's inability to regulate it with insulin, diabetic changes can occur.

One change is the growth of new, fragile blood vessels in the retina of the eye. These vessels can break causing hemorrhages in the eye. That is diabetic retinopathy. Another form of diabetic retinopathy, generally occurring earlier, is the appearance of little red "bubbles" along the retina's capillaries. The appearance of just one bubble is indicative of diabetic retinopathy. There are no symptoms with this condition, hence the importance of a good annual retinal examination by your eye doctor; twice a year is recommended for every diabetic who has had any retinal changes due to the diabetes. If detected, diabetic retinopathy must be immediately treated by an ophthalmologist, probably in conjunction with the physician who is treating your diabetes. Laser surgery is often indicated. Blindness is always a potential danger.

WHAT TO DO

Most important, of course, is that the diabetic must get his or her blood sugar level under control. Besides any medical treatment (insulin injections, oral medication, or other methods) that is required, the diabetic should exercise every day, and should have a very controlled diet. This may not be easy, but it is essential. Foods to avoid include all foods that contain sugar, and foods with processed grains. It is a good idea to become familiar with your choices of whole grains. Pay careful attention to the first ingredient listed on the package—which should be a whole grain. Breads, cereals, and pastas made with whole grains are readily available in health food stores and most supermarkets. Eat brown rice or wild rice rather than white or yellow rice. Aspartame, (Nutrasweet) is not a good sugar substitute either. It is a known eye toxin. Fruit sugar, stevia, and brown rice syrup are good alternatives. All low-fat protein foods are fine, as are most fresh vegetables and fruits. Organic is your best choice.

SUPPLEMENTS

- The most important supplement in dealing with diabetes is a good multi-vitamin and mineral supplement. I always recommend the most complete and absorbable product of its kind on the market that I know of. Remember, most minerals cannot be found in your foods, so a proper supplement is essential.
- Omega-3 capsules and a daily clove of raw garlic, or a garlic tablet as previously described are also recommended supplements along with bilberry, which is found in a good eye specific supplement.

If you are a diabetic and want to do the best that you can to control your diabetes and to prevent diabetic retinopathy and other ravages of diabetes:
1. See your physician as often as instructed, and please follow all of his or her recommendations completely.

2. Check your blood sugar as often as recommended by your physician.
3. Have your eyes examined twice a year once any diabetic changes are observed in the eye.
4. Exercise every day.
5. Follow a strict diet.
6. Take your supplements as recommended.
7. Check with your physician prior to initiating steps 4 through 6 above.

Chapter 6

Styes

There are two types of styes—external stye, or hordeolum, and internal stye, or chalazion. External styes occur on the upper or lower lid margin, and appear as one or more small red pimples. They form at the opening of a tear duct when it gets blocked by makeup or dirt. They also occur from makeup that has become contaminated by bacteria. Styes also develop when you are run down from lack of sleep, anxiety, an illness, or poor nutrition.

An internal stye, or chalazion, generally appears individually and is found within the upper or lower eyelid—not on the lid margin. It feels like a little round stone in the lid. The internal stye is caused by a blockage of a tear duct leading from a gland in the eyelid. The blockage is a result of dried tears. Tears are composed of various oils that can thicken and harden when dry. The tears back up and form a little "ball" inside the lid. If infected, the overlying and underlying lid will be red, tender and swollen.

WHAT TO DO

For external styes and infected internal styes, hot compresses can be applied to the closed eye, or, alternatively, an appropriate antibiotic can be applied. Once the infection is cleared, the hard little "stone" remains, in the case of the internal stye. This can be softened in some instances by rubbing the lid with warm olive oil. If unsuccessful, the chalazion must be removed surgically. This is a simple procedure performed in the doctor's office.

PREVENTION

If you are prone to getting styes, it would be wise every night before bedtime to use a lid scrub, which is an eyelid cleaner and disinfectant. If your body is rundown, a good multivitamin and mineral supplement, as previously described could be extremely helpful.

Chapter 7
Dry Eye

Dry eyes are a common symptom that can affect anyone. They are more prevalent among the aged, contact lens wearers, and people who have undergone LASIK surgery. Women are nine times more prone to dry eyes. It can also accompany rheumatoid arthritis, scleroderma, and systemic lupus. It can be caused by a vitamin A deficiency, and by lowered immune response.[9] Its symptoms include scratchy eyelids on the eyes, red eyes, or blurry vision that clears up with several blinks. Contact lens wearers may find their contacts sticking to their eyes, or else frequently falling out. Moisturizing eye drops tend to help but only for a short period of time.

WHAT TO DO

In addition to using preservative-free moisturizing eye drops as needed, nutritional protocols may be beneficial. These include eliminating common food allergens and processed foods, such as milk, pasteurized dairy products, corn, wheat, and nightshade plants (including tobacco and the drug Motrin which is nightshade-based.) Reduce all re-

---

[9] Page, Linda Rector, N.D., Ph.D., Healthy Healing, Healthy Healing Publications, 1996.

fined sugars, red meats, and saturated fats. Increase the use of cold-water fish in your diet, which will increase your consumption of Omega-3 fish oil. This is found in salmon, codfish, sardines, or trout and should be eaten every day. On any day that fish is not eaten, a 1,000 mg. Omega-3 fish oil capsule should be consumed with food three times a day. If you have difficulty digesting the fish oil or any fat, including animal or dairy fat, also take a lecithin capsule with food three times a day. Lecithin emulsifies, or breaks down the fat, enabling it to be digested and utilized by the cells of the body more easily. If you are allergic to fish or you are a vegetarian, a flax oil capsule, liquid flax oil or ground flax seed can be taken in lieu of the fish oil capsule. For severe dry eyes, a nighttime preservative-free ointment is recommended. Also, consult with your eye doctor. Your doctor might advise procedures and/or medications in addition to the above recommendations. There are many different causes for dry eyes and a professional eye examination is recommended to determine the course of action to be taken.

Chapter 8
Computer Eyestrain

Computer eyestrain, technically known as "Computer Fatigue Syndrome," is a very common problem encountered by people who spend a good deal of time looking at a computer monitor. Symptoms include tired eyes; itchy or burning eyes; red eyes; blurriness; headaches; development of near-sightedness, or increased nearsightedness; generalized fatigue; tightness in neck and shoulder muscles. If you experience one or more of these symptoms, and you spend a good deal of time in front of a monitor, then you have computer fatigue syndrome.

WHAT TO DO

Follow the simple steps that I have outlined below, and you should experience relief of your symptoms:

1. Blink often. Looking at a monitor, one tends to stare. This allows the tears on the eyes to evaporate. Dry eyes tend to get red, itch, and burn. Remember to blink.

2. Periodically, every five or ten minutes, look away from the monitor briefly. You must focus on something that is at least twenty feet away. A clock on

the wall or a sign outside a window is fine. Do not look at just a blank wall. What you are doing is relaxing your eye's focusing muscles. Whenever you look at something that is closer than twenty feet away, you are using your focusing muscles. If you held a fist for a period of time, your arm would tire. That is what happens to your eye muscles. If you open your fist for a few seconds and then tighten up again, you can hold the fist for some time again. The same thing goes for your eye muscles. When they "need a break," they let you know. That is when things start to get blurry, your eyes feel tired, you have difficulty concentrating, or you get a headache. Remember to look away from the monitor on a regular basis. Also, every hour or so, get up and walk around the room or down the hall. This very short break will leave you less tired at the end of the day and more efficient at your work on the computer.

3. Have the monitor at or below eye level; never above. It is much more difficult for you to look up and near than to look down and near. If you can raise your seat or else lower the monitor so that you are looking slightly below eye level, you will reduce your eye fatigue, general fatigue, and shoulder and neck tightness.

4. Do not have a window in front of or behind the monitor; it should be on one side of it. If it is in front of the monitor, you will be facing a source of glare that is tiring on the eyes. If it is behind the

monitor (and you), you will get a reflection of the glare on the monitor, which also causes eyestrain.

5. From where you are seated, you should not be able to see a light source without moving your head. Light should emanate from above, behind, or on the side of you. Also, you should not be able to see a reflection of the light source on the screen of the monitor. That glare is very tiring on the eyes. It also reduces the contrast of what is on the screen of the monitor making it more difficult to see. This too causes eyestrain.

6. A tinted glare-free glass only screen over the monitor is helpful in eliminating stray glare and improving contrast. It also may block the electromagnetic radiation emitted from the monitor. People are affected by this radiation unknowingly, and it is not beneficial to the immune system. If a blocking screen is not available, alternatively wear eyeglasses that have anti-reflection coated lenses with UV block that can be purchased where prescription eyeglasses are sold. A mild reading prescription in the lenses is helpful too for reducing the amount of focusing that your eyes have to do. Many eye doctors are of the opinion that this might help prevent nearsightedness from developing or increasing.

Using flat screen monitors instead of the more familiar cathode ray, low-emitting visual display terminal (VDT), reduces the electromagnetic fields lessening their damaging effects. These may include eyestrain, eye deterioration, and cataracts.[10] Sitting at least 21 inches from a tube-style VDT may also protect you from these fields.[11] Of course, steps one through five must be adhered to as well.

7. If you are over forty years of age, it will be helpful to have the monitor at the same distance as your reading material; about twenty-one inches for a normal stature person. If they are at different distances, one of them will be out of sharp focus unless you keep shifting your viewing distance. This is due to the decrease in focusing ability as we age, and which becomes apparent for most people when they are in their forties. So have your reading prescription eyeglasses made for that distance. It is a good idea to have "computer eyeglasses" which will incorporate a prescription for your working distance, UV block, and an anti-reflection coating. These are then your specialized "work" glasses, just as you might have specialized work clothing or tools. This might help to prevent the development of or the increase in myopia (nearsightedness) common to computer users.

These simple steps should relieve computer eyestrain and provide for a longer, more useful time spent in front of a monitor with less wear and tear on your eyes and your body.

---

[10] Anderson, N., Benoist, A., *Your Health and Your House*, Keats Publishing, 1994.
[11] Ibid.

Chapter 9

Red Eye

Many books have been written about "red eye," and this booklet would not be complete without at least a brief description of it here to acquaint the reader with red eye and to caution the reader as to its possible implications. A red eye does not necessarily mean "pink eye." Pink eye refers to only one type of red eye condition that is otherwise known as acute epidemic conjunctivitis, and it is the most contagious disease known to affect humans.

First, let us look at what a red eye is. The white of the eye (the sclera) is overlaid by a clear protective skin (the conjunctiva) that has many tiny blood vessels. When these blood vessels get engorged due to an irritant, they become visible, and the eye appears red. The underlying sclera has blood vessels too that can become engorged and the eye will appear red. When the blood vessels of the conjunctiva become visible, the condition is known as conjunctivitis. There are many types and causes of conjunctivitis including bacterial, viral, and allergic. Conjunctivitis can also accompany an inflammation elsewhere in the eye.

When your eye is red, it may be a type of conjunctivitis or it may be that another segment of your eye has an involvement that can also cause the redness. Sometimes this can be quite serious, and if not attended to immediately, you might end up with permanent vision loss, or at the worst, blindness. There is not always pain with a red eye, sometimes just a feeling of discomfort or grittiness. Do not be lulled into a false sense of "oh, it's nothing and will clear up soon." A red eye needs to be seen by your eye doctor immediately. Only your doctor can determine whether the red eye is inconsequential or not. Do not put it off another day.

SUMMARY

I have attempted to provide you with a brief insight into some common eye conditions—what they are, and how YOU might prevent them or control their advance. For the most part, this involves regular exercising, eating specific foods while avoiding others, and taking the proper supplements. Quit smoking and avoid second-hand smoke. Regular exercise does not necessarily mean joining a gym. A ten-minute fast walk per day is adequate; a twenty-minute fast walk per day is ideal. The foods and some of the supplements previously recommended are available in local health food stores and supermarkets. The supplements described in this book may be available from your eye care professional. Ask. If you cannot find a convenient outlet for these supplements, you can email me at -mail: pure4us@aol.com and I shall be happy to direct you to one.

Supplement Recommendations List:

- Multi-vitamin and mineral tablet or caplet for people fifty and older and one for under 50.
- Nutritional extracts specific for eye health that include at least lutein, bilberry, quercetin, eyebright, zinc, selenium, Vitamin C, Vitamin E and beta carotene
- Co-enzyme Q10 with vitamin E
- Omega-3 essential fatty acids derived from fish oil (preferred) or else from flax seed
- MSM, which is a purified organic form of sulfur
- Garlic (enteric coated) derived from fresh garlic
- Calcium and magnesium in the most bioavailable chelated form
- Lecithin (from soybeans) supports healthy cellular and metabolic function. Emulsifies fat.
- Ginkgo Biloba (for glaucoma)
- Detoxifying tablet

Index

A-D

E-I

L-N

O-R

S-T

U-Z

Bibliography

-Abel, R., *The Eye Care Revolution,* Kensington Books Pub, New York, NY, 1999.

-Abel, R., Richer, S., Sardi, B., "The Case for Nutrition as Preventive Eye Care," *Review of Optometry,* Aug. 1995.

-American Diabetes Association, On-line, Sept, 2001.

-Anderson, N., Benoist, A., *Your Health and Your House,* Keats Publishing, 1994.

-Anshel, J., *Smart Medicine for Your Eyes,* Avery Publishing, 1999.

-*AREDS,* sponsored by the NEI. "The Effect of Antioxidant Vitamins and Zinc on Age-Related Macular Degeneration and Cataract." Oct. 2001.

-Blumentahl, et al., *Complete German Commission E. Monographs – Therapeutic Guide to Herbal Medicine,* Integrative Medicine Communications in conjunction with American Botanical Council, Boston, MA, 1998.

-Brody,Tom, *Nutritional Biochemistry Second Edition.* San Diego, CA: Academic Press, 1994:621.

-Chan, S., et al., "The role of copper, molybdenum, selenium, and zinc in nutrition and health," *Clinical Laboratory Medicine,* Dec. 1998; 18(4): 673-85.

-Christen, W.G., "Antioxidant vitamins and age-related eye disease," *Proc Assoc Amer Physicians,* 1999; 111:16-21.

-Christopher, John R., *School of Natural Healing Revised and Expanded 20th Anniversary Edition,* Springville, UT.

-Christopher Publications, 434, 1996.

-Eye Disease Case-Control Study Group, "Antioxidant status and neovascular age-related macular degeneration," *Arch Ophthalmol,* 1993; 111:104-9.

-Folkers, K., Shizukuishi, S., Takemura, K., et al., "Increase in levels of IgG in serum of patients treated with coenzyme-Q10 in human blood plasma," *Res Comm Pathol Pharmacol,* 1982; 38:335-38.

-Gerster, H., "Antioxidant vitamins in cataract prevention." *Z.Emahrungswiss,*1989; 28:56-75.

-Gerster, H., "Antioxidant protection of the ageing macula." *Age Ageing,* 1991; 20:60-69.

-Higginbotham, E. J., et al., "The Effect of Caffeine on IOP in Glaucoma Patients." *Ophthalmology,* 1989, 96 (5):624-26.

-*Investigative Ophthalmology* 40: 1477-86, 1999; *Current Eye Research* 20: 215-24, 2000.

-*Investigative Ophthalmology,* ARVO Abstracts 435, B346, 1997.

-Jacques P.F., Chylack L.T., Jr. "Epidemiologic evidence of a role for the antioxidant vitamins and carotenoids in cataract prevention," *Am J Clin Nutr* 1991; 53:352S-55S.

-Jacques, P.F., "The potential preventative effects of vitamins for cataract and age related macular degeneration." *Int J Vitamin Nutr Res,* 1999; 69:198-205.

-Joseph, J., Nadeau, D., Underwood, A., *The Color Code,* Hyperon Books, New York, NY, p. 3, 2002.

-Landrum J.T., Bone, R.A., Joa, H., Kilburn, M.D., Moore L.L., and Sprague K.E., "A one year study of the macular pigment: the effect of 140 days of a lutein supplement," *Exp Eye Res.* 1997; 65:57-62.

-Mowrey, Daniel, B., *The Scientific Validation of Herbal Medicine,* Keats Publishing, New Canaan, CT, 1986.

-Newsome, D.A., Swartz, M., Leona, N.C., Elston, R.C., Miller, E., "Oral Zinc in Macular Degeneration," *Arch Ophthalmol,* 1988, Feb; 106:192-8.

-*Jrnl of the Amer Geriatric Soc.,* 1998, Vol. 46, pp. 1-7.

-*Ophthalmology* 108: 697-704, 2001.

-Packer, Lester, et al., "Antioxidant activity and biologic properties of a procyanidin-rich extract from pine (Pinus maritima) bark, pycnogenol," *Free Radic Biol Med,* Sept, 1999; 27(5-6): 704-24.

-Page, Linda Rector, N.D., Ph.D., *Healthy Healing,* Healthy Healing Publications, 1996.

-*PDR for Nutritional Supplements,* Medical Economics Pub, Montvale, NJ, 2001.

-*Photochemistry Photobiology,* 1999, 70: 353-58.

-Robertson J., Donner A., Trevithick J., "A Possible Role for Vitamins C and E in Cataract Prevention," *Amer J of Clinical Nutr,* Vol. 53 (Suppl), 346S-51S, 1991.

-*Physician's Desk Reference for Herbal Medicines,* First Edition, Medical Economics, Inc., Montvale, NJ, 2001

-Rouhiainen R., Rouhiainen H., Salonen J., "Association Between Low Plasma Vitamin C Concentration and Progression of Early Cortical Lens Opacities," *Amer J of Epidem,* Vol 144, 496-500, 1996.

-Ritch R., *Med Hypotheses.,* 54 (2), 221-35, Feb 2000; Chung H.S., et al. *J Ocular Pharmacol Ther.* 15 (3), 233-40, Jun 1999.

-Saddon, J.M., Ajani, U.A., Sperduto, R.D., Hiller, R., Blair, N., Burton, T.C., Farber, M.D., Gragoudas, E.S., Haller, J., Miller, D.T., Yannuzzi, L.A., and Willett, W., "Dietary carotenoids, vitamins A, C and E, and advanced age-related macular degeneration," *J Am Med Assoc.,* 1994; 272:1413-20.

-Sardi, B., *Nutrition in the Eyes,* Health Spectrum Pub, 1994.

-Sardi, B. "Eradicating Cataracts," *Townsend Letter for Doctors,* June, 1995.

-Schaumberg, I.L., "Vision Problems in the U.S," *Prevent Blindness America, 2000.*

-Seddon, J.M., Ajani, U.A., Sperduto R.D., et al., "Dietary carotenoids, vitamins A,C and E, and advanced age-related macular degeneration." *JAMA*, 1994; 272: 1413-20.

-Seis, H. and Stahl, W., *Lycopene: antioxidant and biological effects and its bioavailability in the human*, Proceedings of the Society for Experimental Biology and Medicine, June 1998: 218(2): 121-4.

-Seis, H., et al., "Antioxidant functions of vitamins, Vitamin E and C, beta-carotene, and other carotenoids," *Annals of the NY Academy of Science*, Sept. 1992: 669: 7-20.

-Snodderly, D.M., "Evidence for protection against age-related macular degeneration by carotenoids and antioxidant vitamins," *Am J Clin Nutr*, 1995; 62(suppl):1448S-61S.

-Taylor, A., Jacques, P.F., et al., "Long-term intake of vitamins and carotenoids and odds of early age-related cortical and posterior subcapsular lens opacities," *Amer J Clin Nutr*, 2002;75(3):540-549.

-Tielsch, Sommer, Witt, Katz and Royall, B"lindness and Visual Impairment in an American Urban Population. The Baltimore Eye Survey," *Arch Ophthalmol*, 1990; 108:286-90.

-Uthus, E.O., and Seaborg, C.D., "Deliberations and evaluations of the approaches, endpoints and paradigms for the dietary recommendations of the other trace elements," *Journal of Nutrition*. Sept. 1996; 126(9 Suppl): 2377-85S.

-Weil, A., "Protect Your Vision Naturally," *Self Healing*, June, 1997, p 2.

-Zand, J., Spreen, A., LaValle, J., *Smart Medicine for Healthier Living*, Avery Penguin Putnam Pub, June 1999: 255.

Other Books by Safe Goods

The Natural Prostate Cure	*$ 6.95 US* *$10.95 CAN*
Natural Born Fatburners	*$14.95 US* *$22.95 CAN*
Lower Cholesterol without Drugs	*$ 6.95 US* *$10.95 CAN*
Macrobiotics for Americans	*$ 7.95 US* *$11.95 CAN*
Cancer Disarmed	*$ 4.95 US* *$ 6.95 CAN*
Dr. Vagnini's Healthy Heart Plan	*$16.95 US* *$24.95 CAN*
Doctor in Your Suitcase	*$ 7.95 US* *$11.95 CAN*
Honey, The Gourmet Medicine	*$ 9.95 US* *$14.95 CAN*
No More Horse Estrogen	*$ 7.95 US* *$11.95 CAN*

For a complete listing of books visit our web site:
www.safegoodspub.com
or call for a free catalog (888) 628-8731
order line: (888) NATURE-1